Why are my clothes shrinking? Addressing Insulin Resistance and Increased Belly Fat.

By Jules Allen-Rowland

This book is dedicated to my sister, Jill

Disclaimer

Medical diagnosis and treatment is constrained by law to be the exclusive monopoly of licensed practitioners. Neither the content, nor the intent of the information in this book, may, or should be construed as the giving of medical advice, nor recommending medical treatment of any kind. This book is for educational purpose only. Reading this book, receipt of information contained in this book, or the transmission of information from this book does not constitute a physician-patient relationship. Always seek the advice of your physician or other qualified health provider with any questions you may have regarding a medical condition. Never disregard professional medical advice or delay seeking it because of something you have read in this book. Always work with a qualified health professional before making any changes to your diet, prescription drug use, lifestyle or exercise activates. The information is provided as-is, and the reader assumes all responsibility for the use, non-use, or misuse of this information.

About The Author

Jules Allen-Rowland, a functional medicine practitioner, writes under her own name, as well as the pen name Maxine Gregg, in the Xpert range. In practice for more than 30 years in the health industry (starting off as a registered podiatrist), Jules has a bachelor's degree in psychology and communication, certification in health, nutrition and exercise science and she added Functional Medicine to round it off. As a registered Functional Medicine Practitioner, she has worked with, or lectured to, more than two thousand patients who struggled with their health and were overwhelmed by the extent of information necessary for negotiating their way towards improved health. Starting the Xpert range has allowed Jules to use her knowledge as a Functional Medicine Practitioner to address serious lifestyle issues in a light-hearted, daybook way, removing the 'weight of change' with regard to health challenges and make them fun and do-able, without compromising the information needed to enjoy lives of vitality and joy. She has written five other books, all in the health and support field.

Taming the Hidden Shrew: How to balance hormones to feel slim, calm and in control. ASIN: B0BFBKPYWS. (Paperback. ASIN: 1776417569)

Get More Lead in Your Pencil. 14 Tips to boost testosterone and last longer in the bedroom. ASIN: B0B9HHTP9S. (Paperback. ASIN: 1776417526)

Ignite Her Fire: What every man needs to know about satisfying women. ASIN: B08FZS4ZF5. (Paperback ASIN: 177641750X)

When are you due? Resolving Gut Sensitivities and Bloating. ASIN: B0BK9KVDQZ (Paperback ASIN: 1776417577)

Where did I leave my keys? How to keep your brain sharp as you age. ASIN: B08NHQ82ZM. Paperback ASIN: 1776417542

Day 1

"Life is 10% what happens to us and 90% how we react to it." – Dennis P. Kimbro

Signs of trouble ahead...

In South Africa where I live, the weather is mostly glorious. Mostly sunny, mostly warm. I find in the heat I am less likely to over- eat but the lure of cool drinks, particularly ice-cold white wine in the early evening, is irresistible. All over, summer bodies are on display but in ever- more stressful lives, coupled with convenience foods, little exercise and higher carbohydrate foods, muffin tops and doughy legs, albeit tanned dough, are becoming more and more prevalent.

To counteract this we search out varied diets and are bombarded with a range of diet options from, - low calorie, - low fat, - low carbohydrate - to banting, as well as constant pressure to exercise until we throw up our hands, give up and have another chocolate or glass of wine. We resolve to try again next week or next month or even next year but for now we squeeze ourselves into our 'diminutive' clothes and just feel uncomfortable and miserable until we are forced to buy a size bigger.

I read a study somewhere that stated that to lose weight I would have to exercise for an hour, five times a week. I laughed: To which hour were they referring? No one I know has another hour to spare in their day and even if I did, I certainly have no plans to use it exercising. I would rather face-time my daughter in the UK.

And yet the obesity and diabetic numbers continue to climb despite access to a wealth of information, now freely available on the internet. Gone are the days when we could claim ignorance as the reason for our poor health. Nowadays I think it is due to information overload, as well as to too little time, that leaves us weak-willed or disinterested in making changes. It is impossible to know where to begin.

But if I was to quantify the most frequent request for help in my practice, it would be to 'lose weight and have more energy' and the two go hand in hand. To top it all, we each know at least one person who suffers from diabetes, and even the diabetics are unsure what food choices to make or what is really going on within the cells, and again, have limited time to read the complex information that come out to explain the intricacies of sugar and insulin management. The quick 15-minute consult at the doctor is also insufficient time to really gain a solid grasp on what is going on in our body, let alone how to resolve it.

I was diagnosed with diabetes at 52 although I suspect that I must have been pre-diabetic for at least 10 years before that, given that I could never lose my belly fat and was always exhausted. My doctor tested my blood sugar every time I saw him, and it was normal, but at that time I didn't know that fasting blood sugar can show as normal for years with underlying insulin imbalances before it finally collapses with everything else. My HbA1C measured 5.7% which I was told was acceptable but all too quickly it shot over the mark to 8.2%. My blood pressure was too high, and I was rubbish at sleeping. I just didn't feel good, never mind look good. Work was hectic and I didn't have time to prepare healthy meals. At the time I always just assumed my body would cope until it just didn't cope any more. Now I realise that managing my stress and taking time out to prepare and enjoy healthy meals is not a luxury but a necessity for life.
Jolene 57

It is hard to face the truth sometimes. Life gives us enough knocks and accepting that we may be on a path to diabetes is easy to overlook. The term ' insulin resistance' is synonymous with pre-diabetes and, even harder to take in is the fact that resistant belly fat is an outward sign of insulin resistance. (A very ugly truth). There is no point in becoming a marathon runner, or cutting calories, if the running is leading to a 'carbo-loading' diet and the reduced calorie foods we eat are foods that increase insulin flood.

I know what I have said may be gobbledegook to you, but I promise by the end of this booklet, you will have an increased understanding that will allow you to make choices that will trim that increasing waistline and reduce your risks of serious, non-communicable diseases.

Signs and symptoms that we may be in trouble are:
- Brain fog
- Exhaustion

- Stubborn belly fat
- Food cravings
- Hungry after dinner
- Midafternoon slump
- Poor sleep patterns
- High triglycerides
- Awakening still tired
- Mood swings

Activity: Tick whether any of the above symptoms apply to you. If they do, you may be starting with insulin imbalance problems

Day 2

"There is no royal road to anything. One thing at a time, all things in succession. That which grows fast, withers as rapidly. That which grows slowly, endures." – Josiah Gilbert Holland

Understanding Insulin...

I have always found that sustainable changes in my life are made more achievable, or in some cases more bearable, when I understand something of the context. While I am not so naive as to think that life is in any way a linear event, in general I have noticed that there are often particular overriding causes that appear to add more weight to change than others, at least in the majority of the cases.

The impact of insulin on many chronic conditions, belly fat and brain fog , is an excellent example.

To understand what has gone awry, it is helpful to compare with what is functioning perfectly and then try and get back to that. What was perfect for your body may not be so for mine. Understanding the delicate hormonal dance that allows our body to manage our energy requirements is first on the list. We have been misguided into thinking that weight loss is about a balance between energy- in versus energy -out.

In other words, when you eat more than you burn, you are going to get fat, and while in some cases this does apply, many overweight people will tell me that they eat hardly anything, and they are still overweight. So what's cutting there? In these cases the web of hormonal and functional processes have been compromised and need to be addressed first and starving ourselves is not a solution. (Thank goodness)

So here goes! For the body to have enough energy to stay alive, our cells need fuel, and the fuel comes in the form of sugars (carbohydrates) and fats. Sugars are the most accessible fuel source, but the body has to somehow get the sugar from the blood into the cells, and this is where insulin comes in.

Insulin is a hormone that not only instructs the body to store energy but is actually the transport for glucose into the cells. Only insulin has the key that will open the cell door to the glucose flowing in our blood from the food we have just eaten. When we eat, our blood glucose rises. The pancreas secretes insulin in response and our insulin level also rises. How much it rises will depend on the amount of sugar (carbohydrate) in the meal as well as what accompanies the carbohydrates. i.e. protein or fat.

Sugar on its own cannot enter the cell. It needs insulin as the key to unlock the cell doors. So insulin picks up the sugar and carries it into the cell and drops it inside. This moves the sugar from the blood into the cell and our blood sugar then returns to normal.

The cell is now able to use the sugar to generate energy (within a little organelle called a mitochondrion) and the cellular glucose level drops as the energy is used.
Now, with lower levels of blood and cellular glucose, we get hungry again and are ready for the next meal.
With no insulin we would die of cellular starvation.

Activity: Take note of how soon after a meal you are hungry again. Are you able to go for 4-5 hours or do you feel cranky and light headed after 2-3 hours.

Day 3

"When I stand before God at the end of my life, I would hope that I would not have a single bit of talent left and could say, I used everything you gave me." – Erma Bombeck

Energy while we sleep...

Of course, as delightful as the idea may seem, we are not ruminants eating all day. We have children to fetch and a career to hold down. Eating is often a quick bite standing at the stove, or a takeaway while we wait for soccer practice to finish. Never mind the fact that a third (we hope) of our day is spent sleeping. So what happens to our energy supply when we are not eating? Our heart still must beat, and our cellular processes turn over and we need energy for that.

Of course, not everyone has a nicely padded bum as a reserve. For me, snarling irritation is the unfortunate side effect when I haven't eaten, but making healthy food choices is not always possible and occasionally I have been caught with nothing but the half-eaten packet of gummy bears in my cubbyhole as the only option to keep insanity at bay.

But the body is remarkable. During the hours when we are not eating our pancreas, instead of producing insulin, will produce a hormone called glucagon, which stimulates the liver into releasing stored glycogen (glycogen is a fancy name for stored sugar), so now instead of the energy source coming from the outside in the form of food, the body pulls it from the liver and muscles, where it has been previously stored. This supply will keep us going while we sleep.
The hormone glucagon also has a very desirable function in that it can stimulates fat burning so when we have burned through our stored glycogen from the liver and muscles, the glucagon will switch to burn fat from our belly or bum. (Sadly there are no glucagon injections to speed up fat loss.)

In a prolonged state of no food coming in, if for example we are sick, glucagon will first stimulate the use of triglycerides from the blood as a quick and ready fuel and then move onto the stored glycogen. This will happen if 4-5 hours have gone with no meal. If we go even longer, it will move on to our stored fats.

In a healthy body, (if you are not insulin resistant), - when the insulin drops after transporting all the glucose and there is no further food supply, the pancreas secretes glucagon.

Glucagon signals the liver to turn the stored glycogen back into glucose as your sugar level begins to drop between meals. It also triggers a process called "gluconeogenesis" which triggers the synthesis of glucose from stored protein and fat. In other words, glucagon is able to actually transform both protein and fat into a fuel our body is able to burn. Normally the body is able to store enough glycogen to keep your body fueled for 24hours of normal activity.

By the time the next meal arrives, provided a suitable amount of time between meals has elapsed, the body will have depleted the glycogen stores and in a normal system, when you eat the next meal, insulin will send about 60% of the calories from the meal back to the liver for storage.

About 40% goes into the muscles for quick access to energy. Insulin will convert a small % of the glucose to fat into the blood. This small increase in the body's fat triggers the release of another hormone called leptin and leptin is the messenger that tells the pancreas it is time to stop producing Insulin. Some insulin is good. Too much is bad.

Activity: Take note of your normal eating patterns. Are you a person who, out of habit, eats 5-6 smaller meals a day? Do you snack just before bedtime? Do you exercise at all?

Day 4

Things going wrong?

In theory of course, I understand the concept of consequences to actions or omissions but in the practical process of living, who amongst us has the time to forever be analysing every morsel we eat or activity we do, or in my case, don't do. I realised I needed to make changes when I turned 40 and my energy bottomed out.

As I had always been a high energy person, I was particularly affected by this because the contrast was so marked. Ironically, despite having no energy, I was also unable to have a good night's sleep. To top it all, my diet was not terrible. So I couldn't attribute the change to fast food.

But a creeping rot was setting in somewhere under my radar. As I have always been someone who enjoys salads, I believed that because I ate salads, I could also eat a substantial amount of chocolate. A burgeoning belly was testament that in my life, something was off balance. So how did things start to go wrong?

1. Firstly, I was eating too often. Upon examination, as well as through experience with hundreds of clients, I have to say that I disagree entirely with advice to eat small meals often, in order to 'balance insulin'. Logically and physiologically, if insulin is a hormone that tells the body to 'store energy' and fat is the way the body stores energy and I was wanting to lose fat, eating often (thus raising my insulin) made no sense at all. Better to limit insulin to the minimum necessary to be a more effective at not storing fat.

Also, in eating often, there was never a deficit of stored energy (glycogen) in the liver and muscles for the incoming calories to replace. It meant that there was never a sufficient break from eating to allow my body to clear out the stored glycogen from the liver and muscles.

Practically what this meant was that if the body stores surplus sugar in the liver and muscles and I never burned that surplus, then any indulgent meal I ate from then on would have no storage place to go except as fat. The liver and muscles were already at full capacity.

2. I did little exercise: Aside from other benefits, doing little exercise meant that the glycogen stored in the muscles was also never burned, leaving no space for the odd surplus treat to store.
Plus, the more toned muscles are, the more glucose they will demand and the more of your calorie intake will go to muscle and not fat.

While I caught this in time, many of my clients have slipped into 'insulin resistance' just through the accumulation of small insults to the body such as eating too often and exercising too little or eating 'diet' foods. (a scourge on health!). As insulin resistance has no sudden and drastic side effects like blindness or an unsightly rash, and it may take 15 years of insulin resistance before becoming diabetes, it is understandable that the slippery slide is missed.

We are also lulled into a false sense of security by repeated glucose tests that come back normal, simply because the more telling tests such as HbA1c or fasting insulin are not done. In short, the continual flow of insulin from your pancreas every time you eat, plus the regular exposure your cells have to insulin, eventually leads to insulin resistance, and eventually tires out the pancreas, increasing your risks of diabetes.

What does it mean to be insulin resistant or early type 2 diabetic?

If you eat frequently, the many meals result in a constant flow of insulin and eventually the cells become insensitive to the insulin. A bit like the way our ears turn off and we no longer hear our children bickering. Insulin, with its package of glucose, is banging on the cell door to be let in and the cells refuse to open.

What is left in the blood is surplus insulin AND the glucose you consumed at the meal that the cells are refusing to allow entry.

The body senses there is still glucose in the blood and releases still more insulin to try and manage the glucose still remaining. Now you have EXTRA insulin, which will then finally drop your blood sugar below normal, leading to something called 'reactive hypoglycemia' and you will feel shaky and weak and starving again, (and irritable) even though you ate enough at the previous meal. It is almost as though all the extra insulin is now demanding glucose so that it has something to do... hence the desire for yet still more food.

Some common signs of Insulin Resistance
- Obesity
- High ratio or middle fat to hip fat
- Hypoglycemia (low blood sugar)
- Metabolic syndrome
- Hypertension (insulin caused kidneys to retain salt)
- Disordered cholesterol ratios. High triglycerides
- PCOS
- Cardiovascular disease

Activity: Have you been diagnosed with metabolic syndrome or Insulin resistance? If not and you suspect you may have a problem because you have some of the signs mentioned, then request an HbA1c and a fasting insulin blood test. believe me they are worth the price. Optimal HbA1c is 4.5% - 5% and optimal fasting insulin is below 5.

Day 5

"When I hear somebody sigh, 'Life is hard,' I am always tempted to ask, 'Compared to what?'" – Sydney Harris

Health problems associated with high insulin...

Accepting that high insulin will make me fat is one thing, but I have noticed that being fat has some aesthetic advantages (yes!) as women who carry a bit more fat look younger than their thin counterparts. Plus, if your hubby or partner doesn't mind you being a bit chubby, why should we care? Why not come to terms with this and just love our bodies as they are?

I applaud the idea of this. I believe that personal acceptance is intensely attractive and contributes to a sense of calm and as I have seen the stress caused by lovely women that are perfectionists, I fully subscribe to accepting and loving our body, but there is a margin at which acceptance needs to be nudged into wellness. I see it time and time again. When we are young, a gorgeously rounded body causes no unpleasant signs and symptoms but when we hit even late 30's and are balancing small children and careers, suddenly our body cannot cope any more.

Sadly there are other conditions that begin to rear their ugly little heads when we have high levels of insulin or are insulin resistant or diabetic.

Why does it matter if I have high insulin
- Prolonged inhibition of fat burning. It just takes longer to lose weight.
- Excess belly fat which is uncomfortable and unsightly.
- Decreased lean muscle mass, so we get weaker.
- Damage to blood vessel linings. Atheroma formation and increased risk of stroke.
- Systemic inflammation, which increases our risk of heart attacks and even cancer.
- High blood pressure.
- Thick blood which increases the strain on the heart.
- Water retention. Weight gain and swollen ankles.

- Initiation of cancer through oxidative damage. This means too many free radicals formed and damaging both our DNA and our cellular functioning.
- Alzheimer's. Called type 3 diabetes because of its association with high blood sugar.
- Thyroid deficiencies and the associated inability to lose weight.

Practical impact in the body
When we have insulin resistance, the increased fat is laid down in the liver and this blocks the steady flow of glycogen we need for when we are not eating. Practically it makes it very hard to go 5-6 hours, or even overnight, with no food, so we begin to need midnight snacks, which further drive up our insulin. This also throws out our leptin levels. Leptin is the hormone that tells the body when we are full and it's time to stop eating. Leptin resistance goes hand in hand with insulin resistance and we no longer get the signal that we can stop eating now!

Plus, excess sugar is very ageing. The sugar lines the inside of the cells, including the blood vessels, and makes them stiff. This ages them faster. (Including your skin cells). Measuring your HbA1c will tell you if you have sugar in your cell wall. (Optimal is between 4.5% and 5%) Higher levels are not desirable as it contributes to an increase in our risk of cardiovascular disease and mental decline.

Activity: Do you have high blood pressure? Measure your blood pressure to check. Many clinics or pharmacies do this for a small fee.

Day 6

"The real opportunity for success lies within the person and not in the job." – Zig Ziglar

Delicious breakfast recipe...

I adore the scent and the flavour of cinnamon. It reminds me of warmth and fireplaces and hot toddy's, but it is also a rather special spice in that it positively affects how the body responds to insulin. There is a phytonutrient contained in cinnamon called MHCP that stimulates the binding capacity of insulin to cells. It mimics insulin and assists the transport of glucose into the cells, which is very helpful when insulin resistant. The bonus is that cinnamon is readily available, cheap, and actually tastes good. Use the ground cinnamon and preferably one that has no gluten.

The following recipe for cinnamon breakfast crunch comes from a delightful site called Gnom-Gnom. I just love the name. The site has wonderful recipes.
https://www.gnom-gnom.com/grain-free-keto-cinnamon-toast-crunch/

Cinnamon Toast Crunch

Ingredients
- 144 g almond flour
- 35 g coconut flour
- 1 teaspoon xanthan gum *
- 3/4 teaspoon baking powder

- 3/4 teaspoon baking soda
- 2 teaspoons cinnamon
- 1/2 teaspoon kosher salt
- 6 tablespoons Swerve **
- 2 teaspoons apple cider vinegar
- 2 teaspoons vanilla extract
- 54 g grass-fed butter cold and diced
- 1 egg lightly beaten

For 'sugar' cinnamon topping:
- 40 g grass-fed butter melted
- 1-2 tablespoons Swerve **
- 2 teaspoons cinnamon

Instructions
- Preheat oven to 350°F/180°C.
- Add almond flour, coconut flour, xanthan gum, baking powder, baking soda, cinnamon, salt, and Swerve to a food processor. Pulse a few times until thoroughly combined.
- Add apple cider vinegar and vanilla extract with food processor running. Once thoroughly combined, add in butter and pulse a couple of times until thoroughly combined and broken up into pea-sized pieces.
- Pour in egg and with the food processor running. Stop once dough comes together into a ball. Wrap the dough in cling film and allow to rest for 10 minutes (very important!).
- Work in batches. Line counter with parchment paper. Turn out half the dough and place another parchment paper (or wax paper) on top and roll it out as thin as you can.
- Using a ruler, cut dough lengthwise and then crosswise. Prick each piece with a small fork.

- Transfer parchment paper with the cinnamon toast crunch to a baking sheet or tray. Bake for 4 minutes, remove from oven, brush with melted butter and sprinkle with cinnamon sugar. Return to oven for 6-8 more minutes. As each oven is different, watch out after minute 8 for excessive browning (ours is ready at minute 11).
- Transfer to a rack straight away to avoid continued browning.
- Allow to cool completely before enjoying, as they will crisp up when cooling. Once cool, break the pieces apart and store in an airtight container for up to 5 days. Do note that you can always freeze part of the dough, allowing it to thaw completely in the fridge before using.

And if by any reason your cereal won't crunch up (humidity or varying flours): turn on your oven, let the temperature reach 350°F/180°C, turn it off, pop your trays with the cereal back inside, and leave them there for 20 minutes. They'll be sure to dry out and crunch up after cooled.

Recipe Notes
*If Paleo, substitute the xanthan gum for 1 tablespoon ground flax seeds. Just note that the dough will be slightly more fragile than with xanthan gum. And, if preferred, use coconut oil instead of the grass-fed butter.
DO NOT use psyllium husk here, as it helps baked goods retain moisture (and your cereal won't be crunchy!).

Activity: Breakfast is often a difficult meal to plan for. Make and store this crunch for when you need a quick, 'low insulin impact' breakfast.

Day 7

"Luck is a dividend of sweat. The more you sweat, the luckier you get." – Ray Kroc

How stress impacts on insulin...

I am going to harp back to stress management again here. In fact by the end of this book you will be so bored of the words 'stress management' I hope you will address it just to shut me up.

Stress is counter- productive when you want to lose weight and be healthy. It is a massive block to all the roads to health and it frustrates me senseless because we live in a world where stress is inevitable and getting worse. The vicious cycle of demanding jobs, children, poor sleep patterns, exposure to damaging foods, electromagnetic radiation from cell phone towers, low nutrient intake and other factors kick us into a never-ending cycle of stress that our poor body has to deal with, sometimes on an hourly basis, and our body gets fatter as a result.

When we encounter a stressful event, (in the old days it was running from a saber-toothed tiger. Now it is dealing with a demanding boss, or a two-year-old) our body appropriately releases our stress hormones, namely adrenalin and cortisol.

This is good. (At least for that moment). It allows us to focus on dealing with the emergency and one of the ways it does this is to trigger a release of the stored sugar (from our liver and muscles) into the blood so that we have an immediate energy source if we need to run away.

But as described above, when there is sugar in the blood, the body will release insulin to take it into the cells. Of course in nature, when you have run madly, you will burn all that excess but in today's world, exposed as we are to chronic stress, the body doesn't know the difference and continues to flood out cortisol, with the accompanying insulin elevation. In effect we are having a snack every time we deal with a stressful event. Of course we will get fat or be unable to lose weight with this vicious cycle.

In addition, if we eat foods that are low in nutrients, we have insufficient vitamins and minerals to promote cellular management of this stress response and this makes it worse and adds to the stress load that the body has to deal with, digging us deeper into the pit. Too much stress = too much insulin=insulin resistance.

Managing stress is paramount. First on the list is getting enough sleep, but failing that, I have found just 10 minutes a day meditating or quietly resting my mind recharges me. A quick and easy stress reduction you can do several times a day is belly breathing. Set a ping on your phone hourly, or every time you go to the bathroom, stay seated for a bit longer and breathe.

How to Belly Breathe
- Find a comfortable place to sit or even lie down. Place one hand on your abdomen, over the navel, and the other hand on your chest.
- Gently breathe out and then inhale slowly through your nose, counting to 4, pushing out your abdomen slightly and concentrating on your breath. Feel the hand over your abdomen move out as you breathe in. Hold the breath for a count of at least 4 or 5 but remain comfortable. Do not force the process.

- Slowly exhale through your mouth while counting to 6. Gently contract your abdominal muscles to completely release the remaining air in the lungs.
- Concentrate on keeping shoulders relaxed during the process.
- Repeat a few times. You may be able to do only 1 or 2 cycles at first.
- Once you feel comfortable with your ability to breathe into the abdomen, it is not necessary to use your hands on your abdomen and chest.

Activity: Set a reminder on your phone and belly breathe 2-3 rotations when the reminder pings. You can even do it driving but don't close your eyes of course. :)

Day 8

"When I let go of what I am, I become what I might be." – Lao Tzu

Am I insulin resistant?

A good way to see if you have insulin resistance is to walk towards a wall. If your tummy touches the wall first then you can be pretty certain you have a degree of insulin resistance.

I didn't much like this definition because I know how easy it is for this tummy state to creep up on us, but I was reading a very insightful book by Jordan Petersen called 12 Rules for Life: An Antidote to Chaos, and he observed that most people take more care of their pets than they do of themselves.

I was astounded when I read that because I too have noticed that people will spend thousands at the vet when their dog is looking listless, cook fresh food daily for the animal (yet refuse to assemble a salad for themselves), force the prescribed vitamins down the throat of a large bull-mastive twice daily, yet forget to take their own vitamins when the bottle is in full view on the breakfast table and all they need to do is extend an arm and of course, if they know something is bad for the animal, like xylitol is for dogs, in some cases refuse to even keep it in the house in case the dog gets hold of it by mistake.

Yet, the most frequent excuse I hear when I address even overt food sensitivities in my patients is, 'My doctor says I can eat this as long as it's in moderation.' They would never give their dog moderate amounts of chocolate knowing dogs and chocolate don't mix. Paradoxically we care more for our animals than for ourselves.

It is crushing to hear that a treat we adore is now no longer on the menu and if we suspect we have insulin resistance, to begin resolving it we need to look at all contributing causes.

Other factors that may cause Insulin resistance.
- Genetic predisposition:
- Omega 6:3 ratio or trans fats in cell membrane. We need more omega 3 to make the cell membranes receptive to insulin
- Deficiencies of chromium, magnesium, zinc, B-vitamins. All help in insulin management.
- Lack of exercise.
- Excessive sugar, processed foods, starches, fruit juices, and soda
- Stress because it increases cortisol and cortisol causes a release of sugar from the liver and muscles
- Insufficient protein or protein malabsorption

- 6 Small meals a day

Activity: Tick off on the list above any possible causes of Insulin Resistance you may have.

Day 9

"You may find the worst enemy or best friend in yourself." –
English Proverb

Getting good quality sleep...

Sleep is restorative. Particularly in a bedroom that you have created as your sanctuary and your joy. Without a delicious 7-8 hours of sleep at night, problems take on a malevolence that kicks us further into a downward spiral. Our ability to manage conflict, our job, our relationship and even activities and hobbies we may have enjoyed in the past, become challenges we need to overcome. Stress levels climb (did I just use that word 'stress' again?), cortisol flows and of course, as soon as cortisol rises, our body reads this as 'Sabre-tooth tiger stress' and sugar flows into the blood from the muscles, to prepare us to run.

Eating, eating, all the time! Insulin flows and we get fatter with more brain fog.

Sleep should not be a secondary luxury only indulged in after we have finished a quick report, fed the family, tidied the house, and put the plates in the dishwasher and then, because 'me time' is so precious, lost ourselves in a book for an hour. A day that only finishes after 10.30 is detrimental to our health and our waistline.

It is in the nature of many women to put our needs second, third, or even fourth. There is a deep satisfaction in being the parent our child calls for in the middle of the night and there is satisfaction in feeling needed. Of course, for some single mothers there is no fallback assistance from a spouse, so we have to just get on with it, but for these brave and resilient women there has to be another plan that allows us to sleep properly a few nights a week. Asking for help is not a sign of weakness. It is common sense in the face of so many sleep robbers and health obstacles.

I read somewhere about an international organization called 'The Trusted House Sitters'. How fabulous if a similar closed and area bound organization could arise, where mommies could get together and share in the baby-sitting duties. For one night a week, your home becomes the home for 3 other children and their mommies get the night off.

Similarly your children spend the night with another mommy another night and you get to have a deep, scented bubble bath, read a book, go to bed early and *sleep.* Why do we find the concept of farming our children off for a night and having 'me time' distasteful?

I suspect it has less to do with thinking we are being irresponsible (because we can perform the right safety and security checks) than never wanting to 'not' be the centre of our child's world.

Adding people who can love our child and who our child can interact with, is healthy. Other caregivers do not have to be the same as us. 'Different' is good, as long as our children are happy and safe. (And most children find a new environment and new toys fascinating). Adding two children -not your own- to your brood once a week is really worth getting 2 nights off a week. We are not being bad mothers to want health time for ourselves and getting restorative sleep is more than just health time. It is essential to our future survival, our risks of diabetes, Alzheimer's, dementia, heart disease and cancer.

A good night's sleep is the single most impactful health habit we can develop that encompasses reducing our risk of contracting all the non-communicative chronic diseases. (This and cutting out sugar). Don't feel guilty about planning everything you can to get a good night's sleep.

Activity: List anything you can think of that prevents you from getting a good night's sleep. Next to each obstacle try and add at least one solution. Have a 'think tank tea party' with your friends to help come up with ideas.
List the number of people you know from family to friends, to other school mothers, who may be in the same boat as you with regard to obstacles to sleep. Decide whether you can help each other.

Day 10

"Whoever loves much, performs much, and can accomplish much, and what is done in love is done well." – Vincent Van Gogh

---

Bringing insulin down...

Accepting that we may be insulin resistant is tantamount to accepting that we may be an alcoholic. It strikes like a sharp knife, right into the gut and our heart squeezes with fear, because facing a health challenge and giving voice to it, means we are now forced to do something about it or succumb to one of the chronic diseases the condition may portend. Ignorance is much more soothing.

But if, upon reflection, (and ticking too many of the ghastly little boxes), you decide you may be at risk, then of course a plan of action to mitigate the risks is advisable.
None of us wants to change our comfortable habits. This is understandable and in fact, many of our habits help to reduce our level of stress because automatic behavior frees up our mind to other, more mentally demanding activities. Imagine if we needed to think through every little action in our day? We would burn out before long.

How do I bring my insulin down?

- **Don't smoke.** Nicotine enhances the breakdown of fats and increases the delivery of the fats to the liver. This increases the fat laid down in the liver and the increased fat blocks the flow of glycogen out the liver when we are not eating. This results in more need to have midnight snacks and an inability to go long hours between meals.
- **Lose weight.** Hah! Easier said than done, but excess body fat causes leptin resistance. Leptin is the hormone that tells the body when we are full so we can stop eating. When we have leptin resistance, there is enough leptin because leptin is manufactured by fat cells but the message that we are full is not being heard. So we eat more because we feel hungry.
- **Change your diet/ supplements.** Mmmm... ok, we know this but what do we change and what supplements do we add or take away. (More about that later)
- **Exercise:** Exercise clears the stored glycogen from the muscles so the body can dump excess in the space created. This allows any excess sugar in the blood to be pulled back into the muscles for storage and when the blood glucose diminishes, so too does the need for insulin. With reduced insulin the cells are able to re-sensitise.
- **Manage Stress.** That word again!
- **Drink Water.** This is an indirect approach. When we are properly hydrated we are less hungry and less likely to snack so remember to place that jug of water in sight and drink often. Often the sensation of hunger is actually the sensation of thirst and goes away after drinking.

Activity: Take special care to drink enough water.

Day 11

"Courage is the first of human qualities because it is the quality which guarantees all others." – Winston Churchill

Important supplements for addressing high insulin...

I don't much like pills. I went through a patch while I was turning my own health around when I was taking a handful of supplements. I reckon I could probably have dispensed entirely with breakfast because the cellulose enclosing my multitude of capsules would have sufficed but I felt better as a result of them. I was making food transitions at the time and to source organic was another chore that added to the load. In South Africa where I live, unless you grow your own veggies, organic is not readily available.

First prize for health is always to eat the right foods but sadly food nowadays is depleted of vitamins and minerals. If you are healthy this poses no problem but if you are needing to address certain health problems, then supplements are unavoidable.

Taking the correct supplement for your concerns is important, as hit and miss is just a waste of money and to coin a term I have heard often... 'Just makes expensive urine'.

This term is actually true of prescribed medicines as well as nutrient rich food, if your body is not able to digest properly: and as we grow older, our digestive enzyme become less effective. Added to that, many people who are highly stressed are on proton pump inhibitors as well as over the counter ant-acids. The result of these is reduced digestive ability.

While this appears desirable if we have heart burn or reflux, in actual fact reduced digestion has long-term ramifications on our health status. Taking supplements without good gut function, (either as a result of age or stress or medication) is indeed a waste of money but let's assume we have addressed our gut as per 'So, when are you due? (Another Xpert publication) and want now to address our insulin resistance. What do we need to take?

The three essential supplements are magnesium, chromium and omega3.

Magnesium: Excess insulin (as in insulin resistance) has an unfortunate effect on magnesium. It causes magnesium to be excreted more rapidly. But ironically, for insulin to bind properly to the insulin receptor, the receptor needs magnesium to keep it intact. This creates a vicious cycle. How does magnesium support insulin? Imagine you are in a small space ship, and you need to dock on the Star ship Enterprise. The docking station needs to be a perfect fit for your ship. Magnesium ensures the perfect fit on the Star Ship (the cell) for your ship (insulin)
The vicious cycle between insulin resistance causing increased loss of magnesium, and deficient levels of magnesium leading to insulin resistance, is a double whammy.
This is one of those instances when a supplement is necessary. The dosage should be 600mg -800mg.

Testing magnesium is a good idea. Please test red blood cell magnesium (RBC) and not serum. Testing serum magnesium is a waste of time. Optimal levels should be around 2.5mmol/1

Chromium: Chromium Polynicotinate is best. It is stored in the liver and when insulin is released so is chromium, to help with the efficiency of insulin binding to the cells. As with magnesium, when insulin is chronically elevated it forces chromium to be excreted.
If you have insulin resistance, supplement with between 800mcg and 1000mcg per day. Avoid taking it at night because it may keep you awake.

Some of my patients tell me that it blunts their sugar cravings (Bring it on!) so take it at those times in the day when you know you will start to dream of tea and biscuits.

Omega 3: Amongst other wonderful health benefits discussed later, omega 3 improves the integrity of the fatty cellular membrane through which the insulin carrying the glucose has to pass. Optimal dosage is 1000-2000mg of combined EPA and DHA.

Activity: Source and purchase magnesium, omega 3 and chromium. Remember that magnesium may give you a runny tummy in which case go for Magnesium Glycinate, but magnesium citrate is also good. Chromium comes as chromium picolinate and polynicotinate versions. I prefer the polynicotinate form. Omega 3 may be contaminated with mercury so choose a reputable supplier.

Day 12

"The great thing in this world is not so much where you stand, as in what direction you are moving." – Oliver Wendell Holmes

Understanding Glycaemic Index versus Glycaemic Load...

Let's inject some practical steps into the understanding of insulin in the body. If eating carbohydrates stimulates the release of insulin and the amount released is commensurate with the amount of glucose released from the food, then it follows that reducing the amount of high sugary foods is advisable. But how can we recognise what is a food that will release more sugar compared with one that releases less?

This is explained in the difference between High GI foods and High GL foods

GL and GI are numbers that reflect the impact that a particular food has on the amount of sugar in the blood.
The higher the number of the Glycemic Index, (GI) the quicker the rise of sugar in the blood. Table sugar, for example, causes a fast rise in blood sugar. Similarly white bread. Even though bread does not taste sweet, it is a simple carbohydrate with no fiber, and it takes no time at all for the body to break it down into pure glucose. Potato is another carbohydrate that breaks down very fast.

A quick summary.

Whenever there is a rise in blood sugar, the pancreas will secrete insulin and while limited insulin is necessary, too much insulin causes insulin resistance and increases risks of diabetes.

There are many helpful Apps that will tell you the GI and the GL of the foods you want to eat. Foods with a GI greater than 45 are best avoided, especially if one is overweight or diabetic. In fact, for long term health, even slim people should stick to foods with a low GI, but the good news is , some foods, although high GI, are also high in fiber or water, so in normal portion sizes, have very little impact on the sugar in the blood. An example of this is carrot. It takes 6.6 cups of carrots to impact on blood sugar in the same way as 1 cup of cooked spaghetti. Strawberries, for example, have a glycemic index (GI) of 40 but a glycemic load (GL) of 3.6.

The glycemic load takes this into consideration and is thus a more practical measure of what impact the carbohydrate is having in the body.
A rule of thumb is Vegetables and salads are low in GL because they have lots of fibre. Fruit is high in GL because it has a high fructose content and ready sugars. When you want to minimise the insulin flood, stay away from fruit as well as any breads, biscuits and even butternut and beetroot. Even though fruit is full of anti-oxidants, it is bad for insulin release.

Just a little sneak trick. You can bring down the GL impact by eating the food you are craving with fat and protein or add avocado.

Activity: If you have some foods you love and eat often, look up their GL and record it. If you have insulin resistance it may be advisable to stay away from them until you resolve the insulin resistance. Fruit is not always good for everyone.

Day 13

"Live each day as if your life had just begun." – Johann Wolfgang Von Goethe

Avoiding the blame game...

My mother, a very practical and wise woman, offered sage advice with pretty much every momentous happening in my drama filled teenage years (my drama even crept into my early 20's) , 'Never play the blame game.'

While the maxim has been valuable when fighting with my closest friend, or even with my husband, I have realised that even when I am extrapolating information I have received from a scientific study into a plan of action in treating a patient, for every one study I read, citing a cause for a condition, I will find another study either refuting that or offering an alternative cause. It can become complicated excavating the true cause for any one person's condition and the inclination to attach blame to the person for doing 'something wrong' is tempting.

While being overweight is often a factor in insulin resistance and type 2 diabetes and offering solutions to lose weight and change the trigger for insulin release is helpful, there are other, sometimes hidden factors that we have little control over, that may also play a role in insulin resistance, particularly whether or not our insulin resistance becomes diabetes.

Type 2 diabetes is, in part, a lifestyle disease but it develops as a result of a combination of factors, of which poor food choices is only one.
In other words, if you get type 2 diabetes, it is not always your fault, as is commonly suggested by the media.

An interesting study showed that people who are overweight and insulin resistant, who had little exposure to persistent organic pollutants(POP's), never developed diabetes no matter how overweight they became or how insulin resistant they were, whereas those who were exposed to high levels of POP's, did develop diabetes.

Similarly, there are thin people, or even muscular, active people, who have insulin resistance and go on to develop diabetes because they have been unfortunate enough to inherit polymorphisms (SNP's) that result in poor insulin management and lousy carbohydrate metabolism.

What this reminds me, is that there is never a linear cause for any condition. The body is a web and the many strands leading to the centre of the web are all interconnected. A touch on one strand will cause the whole web to tremble.
This is both positive and negative in its effect. Positive, because in many cases, one positive change in habit will affect the whole web positively. Similarly, one bad habit may also have a negative ripple effect throughout the whole body. (Smoking, for example)

Persistent organic pollutants (organic compounds that are resistant to environmental degradation), are ubiquitous and extremely difficult to ferret out and eradicate and yet they have a pervasive negative effect on our health.

Factors that influence contracting Type 2 diabetes are:

- Genetics. Gene SNP's such as FTO,TCF7L2 or PPARG (to mention only a few), affect how our body manages carbohydrates. Some genes also affect insulin secretion and not insulin resistance.
- Circadian Rhythm. There is a gene called CLOCK that influences our circadian rhythm, but so does poor sleep habits: for example: not enough bright morning light as well as too much blue light in the evening.
- Gestational diabetes.
- Low birth weight.
- Persistent organic pollutants such as pesticides.
- BPA , phthalates, and other plasticizers. Plastic water bottles, babies bottles, the lining of cans, are all examples of products that contain BPA. We will address this in a later month.
- Arsenic (really????) from our chickens. Arsenic is found in chicken feed because it promotes growth.
- Some prescription medicines: Certain anti-depressants, statins, and anti - hypertensives increase obesity and indirectly, as well as directly, increase risk of Type 2 diabetes.

While it is possible to eliminate many of the factors that increase risk, the hidden ones elude us but making changes where we have the power to do so and taking the firm stance that we will educate ourselves where it matters and look squarely at all information, even that which makes us uncomfortable, is a powerful step. The internet is an accessible tool at our disposal to reference and investigate and we are fortunate to have it.

Activity:1. Buy glass water bottles and bring filtered water from home wherever you go. Drink only from glass. Write down where you eat or drink from containers that have plastic.

2. Make soups and other meals from scratch. Avoid or limit food coming from a can.

Day 14

"Either you run the day, or the day runs you." – Jim Rohn

How important is enough protein?

While we are sleeping, our body is madly busy with the necessary repair from our daily wear and tear. Our metabolic processes are doing their thing, housekeeping within our cells. Sweeping floors and cleaning windows and replacing the putty in the window frames :) but to do this, our body needs raw materials and amino acids (building blocks) from protein are the raw materials needed.

Protein intake is so varied that it is hard to quantify whether we eat too much or too little. It is my observation that elderly people eat too little. Probably because their digestive enzymes are ineffective and they find it harder to digest food and feel discomfort more readily but also because unless one is in a small minority, protein is the most expensive part of the meal and money is tight when on pension. Often with working people, all the protein is consumed at the evening meal, with a high carbohydrate cereal breakfast (convenient in morning rush) and a snacky type lunch.

As all our enzymes, hormones, muscle mass, and even our neurotransmitters, are constructed from amino acids (protein building blocks) we need to have sufficient protein for these processes and the body responds better with smaller pulses over 3 meals a day. Rather than a large steak at night.
Plus, protein at each meal blunts the impact of the carbohydrate portion and this reduces the insulin spike.

Protein for breakfast is of particular importance to our wellbeing.
In order to get us out and about after sleeping, our body secretes its highest does of cortisol in the morning. This bolus of cortisol is like an espresso to our body. Bam! We are awake. (Or we should be). But to make cortisol our body needs protein.
Fortunately we have a ready source in our organs and muscles so the body will take what it needs but it then has to be replaced. Protein at breakfast will replace what is used.

Leptin and insulin are also more balanced later in the day when the body has had a protein heavy breakfast. The traditional breakfast of cereal, muffins, pancakes and even oats are all carbohydrate heavy and result in a glucose spike that requires a concurrent insulin spike. Plus, have you noticed that when you have a carbohydrate breakfast you are starving by mid-morning?

Glucagon, that fabulous and desirable hormone (that I wish came in injectable form because it is our fat burning hormone), is also made from protein.
The protein for breakfast can come in any form and it is beneficial to have at least 1/3 of your daily requirement at breakfast. Generally the optimal amount of protein we need to function well is 1g per kg of our lean body mass and 1.3g/kg if you are over 60 or an athlete.

This means, if your ideal weight is 60kg, and you are doing some exercise, allow for a total daily protein intake of 60g protein of which 20g should be taken for breakfast.

To calculate the protein in your food there are many useful Apps. I like Cronometer. *https://cronometer.com/* But to give you a ball park: 1 egg contains around 7g of protein

Other sources of protein
- Protein powder in smoothie
- Nuts or nut butters
- Lentils
- Piece of chicken
- Leftover stew from dinner

Activity: Google 'Cronometer' and enter the breakfasts you habitually eat. Make a few changes that you feel comfortable with and that will ensure you are having 1/3 of your protein intake at that early meal. I like to add something fresh and raw that has colour for the antioxidants, perhaps chopped tomato and apple.

Day 15

"The difference between a successful person and others is not lack of strength not a lack of knowledge but rather a lack of will." – Vince Lombardi

Breakfast choices...

I am a big fan of soft-boiled eggs. This breakfast reminds me of toddler food, when I could barely see above the edge of the table to dip my soldiers into the egg. It is only now I can appreciate the health in the eggs (rich in choline), and I use gluten free bread. Two eggs, a small slice of GF bread with macadamia nut butter (or avocado) and a few raspberries for colour fills me up till lunchtime but when I don't have time to cook then I have health granola from Gnom-Gnom. Deeelicious!

https://www.gnom-gnom.com/top-secret-grain-free-keto-granola/

Ingredients
- For the keto granola
- 105 g almonds lightly toasted*
- 95 g pecans
- 75 g sunflower seeds lightly toasted*
- 60 g pumpkin seeds lightly toasted*
- 110 g **chia seeds**
- 56 g flax seeds
- 60 g **sesame seeds** lightly toasted
- 8-10 tablespoons **Swerve** or xylitol (we use 8)
- 1 1/2 teaspoon **blackstrap molasses** optional**
- 1/2 teaspoon **cinnamon**
- 2 egg whites
- pink Himalayan salt to taste

Serving suggestions
- almond milk ice cold!
- full-fat Greek style yogurt
- raspberries
- strawberries

Instructions

- Preheat oven to 250°F/120°C. Line a rimmed baking tray with parchment paper.
- Mix almonds, pecans, sunflower seeds, pumpkin seeds, chia seeds and flax seeds in a large bowl. Set aside.
- Lightly toast sesame seeds over medium/low heat for 4 to 6 minutes. Watch out they do not burn, or they'll taste bitter! You know they're ready when they're lightly golden, and you press one between your fingertips and it turns to powder.
- Add sesame seeds, Swerve, molasses (optional) and cinnamon to a food processor and pulse a couple times until powdered and mixed thoroughly.
- Add sesame sugar to nut mix and combine thoroughly. Set aside
- Beat egg whites with an electric mixer until soft peaks form. Fold gently into granola mix until fully combined.

Spread granola onto prepared baking tray in a single layer and sprinkle with pink Himalayan salt. Bake for 45-50 minutes, until they begin to harden, checking every 15 minutes or so. Allow to cool completely, as they'll continue to crisp up while cooling. These also get even crunchier overnight.

Break up in chunks and store in an airtight container for up to a week, in the fridge for 2, or in the freezer for up to 2 months.

Activity: Google a few gluten free and high protein breakfast choices

Day 16

Making some sacrifices...

Most people, including myself, resist being told to give something up. Particularly if that something is as satisfying as the carb laden comfort foods we enjoy so much. Macaroni cheese and pizza! So delicious, filling and satisfying and so horrendous for our padded tummies and our insulin response.

There is no doubt that a salad just doesn't appeal in the same way and yet to achieve our goal, somehow we need to incorporate acceptable changes into our life and trust that as we progress down the road, the cravings for comfort foods will leave us. And they do!

I have first -hand experience of this and although it took me 18 months, I can go to a pizza restaurant with friends and order a salad and watch them devour fragrant pizza and feel nothing. Not even regret.
But I started somewhere with easy steps, and these are my easy steps. I hope they will help you as well.

- No more fruit juice, canned sodas, or juice concentrates. This was an over- night decision for me. I decided that if I wanted to have that piece of chocolate cake I could not do both and I wanted the cake more. I stopped drinking my calories.

- I made a decision that I would eat food that actually looked like food. No processed food that arrived in a box. This meant no more cereals, bought cookies, processed cheese or meat. It meant if I wanted biscuits I had to make them from scratch which was good because I didn't have time to do that every day.
- No take aways. I allowed myself a once a month treat.
- No heated processed or trans fats. If I want hot chips, I made them at home.
- I allow myself one sweet treat a day. This is occasionally a sugary fruit, like mango and occasionally a chocolate. But it certainly is not: fruit for breakfast, biscuits for tea and dessert after dinner. Waaay too much sugar!

Activity: Write a list of 3 items that, from today, you will give up entirely

Day 17

"Don't worry about failures, worry about the chances you miss when you don't even try." – Jack Canfield

More scientific control on glucose...

If you have only a bit of tweaking and pulling to get your health right then it's not necessary to make big changes from the start but if you are very overweight or are struggling with extreme exhaustion, then more extreme measures are necessary. If you have been to your doctor and have had your HbA1c tested and it is over 5.5%, then I recommend you get into a program that calls for tighter controls.

Although testing fasting insulin requires a blood test, it is possible and very easy to measure your own progress at home by measuring your blood sugar using a glucometer (a little machine for measuring the sugar in your blood). A glucometer is a machine you can purchase over the counter and is usually inexpensive. You will need to get testing strips as well. Initially you will need lots of strips while you gather information about what foods kick your blood sugar up and what foods you can eat. People differ and although there are some general guidelines, some foods react badly in certain people.

Draw up a chart as below. Every day, record your blood sugars upon wakeup and after every meal.

	Wake up	Breakfast Foods	1 Hr	2 Hr	Lunch Foods	1 Hr	2 Hr	Dinner Foods
Mon								
Tues								
Wed								
Thur								
Fri								

S a t								
S u n								

As a basic guideline.
- Blood sugar should stay below 6mmol/l and return to 6mmol/l by 2 hours after a meal
- It should never go above 7.7mmol/l no matter what you eat
- Optimal health levels rarely go above 5.5mmol/l
- Avoid foods that take it to above 6mmol/l
- Normal fasting blood sugar is 4.6mmol/l or even below
- When you begin, don't be surprised if your blood sugar is nothing like the guidelines.
- Don't despair. Begin implementing the changes and take note of the meals where your sugar is lower. Repeat those meals and stop eating the foods that spike your blood sugar.
- Initially you will use lots of strips. This is fine. It's money well spent and will save you a fortune in doctor's bills down the line.

Activity: Source and purchase a glucometer and begin testing and recording your food response

Day 18

"Though no one can go back and make a brand-new start, anyone can start from now and make a brand-new ending."
– Carl Bard

An overview of changes...

The only way to measure our progress is to test and see. We are each unique beings and our body has a unique response. This is why a diet that your best friend went on where she lost 5kg may not work at all for you. Knowledge, although sometimes scary, is very powerful because it shows us 'what is' and prevents us from fooling ourselves in our comfort zone of ignorance.

So let's say you are determined this time to succeed in turning your health around, or even just getting rid of your muffin top and you have purchased your glucometer and nearly had a stroke at the readings because they show your blood sugars are way over the top. What can you do about it?

- Cut out all bread, biscuits, sugar, and cold drinks
- Dramatically reduce fruit until you are in control of weight
- Always eat protein for breakfast (and at every meal)
- Eat 2-3 meals a day and do not snack at all.
- Wait 3 hours after dinner before sleeping.
- Go a minimum of 12 hours between dinner and breakfast.

I want to emphasis a particular point here and this is: To re-sensitize the insulin resistant cells to insulin again you have to give them a break from insulin and the only way to do this is to stop eating for long enough stretches so that insulin is cleared from the blood. Eating 5-6 meals a day means that every single time you eat, or snack, your pancreas is releasing insulin. So many meals means that your insulin is elevated the whole day.

Insulin is a hormone and the message it gives the body is *'Store energy'*. As long as you have excess insulin in the blood, you will never burn an ounce of fat and even a tiny morsel, nibbled on between meals, will be stored under the direction of insulin. Eating 5-6 meals a day results in a constant flow of insulin bathing the cells. How can they possible re-sensitize in this wash of 'energy-storing' message? Cells just turn down the dial and stop hearing the message.

The result of this is also a state of nutrient starvation even when we do eat, as the cell receptors just shut down to allowing insulin (and the attached glucose), into the interior of the cell.

Try and go 4-5 hours between meals. Initially you may not manage because the excess insulin in the blood screams out for food. We need to train our cells, like bootcamp, to go longer without food, without crashing and the only way to do this is to feed them highly nutrient dense veggies, salads, protein, and good fats at the actual meal times.

If you find that you eat a meal and you can only go 3 hours till you want to chew your own arm off, then eat some nuts or avocado and the next day, eat more veggies (fibre), and good fats at the meal before the hunger time and see whether you can go longer. Three meals a day of high-quality food should help you manage the in-between times. If you are very hungry between meals, have a cup of tea but instead of adding milk, add a teaspoon of coconut oil or MCT oil. This is very effective in blunting the munchies.

Activity: Track your food and food-response for a week. List what you eat and how long you feel sustained on that meal. You should not feel bad. No weak or shaky feeling. Eat if you feel bad and the next day, change that meal a bit and then see how long you can go. Aim for 4-5 hours NO food, or even milk in your tea.

Day 19

"Life has two rules: #1 Never quit #2 Always remember rule # 1." – Unknown

Slimming while we sleep!

There is nothing so soothing as a cup of tea before bed and for me, what goes with tea like peas go with carrots, are biccies. Crunchy and sweet. Rusks work too:... but sadly, a snack before bed is very damaging to insulin cycles. It messes with your sleep, and it most definitely messes with your glucagon release. Slimming while we sleep means changing this pattern of a before-bed snack. (If you do wake up regularly at 3am and cannot sleep, then have the tea and MCT oil before you sleep)

It takes approximately 2 hours for your blood sugar and its accompanying insulin to return to normal after a meal. (If you have a glucometer then check it for yourself.) Measure your blood sugar before you eat, after you have gone the 4-5 hours no food, eat and then, 2 hours after, measure your blood sugar again. It should be back to fasting state.

As the pancreas does not secrete glucagon and insulin at the same time and we want to get into a fat burning state while we are doing nothing so strenuous as turning over in our beds, we need to be depleted of insulin before bed time. Glucagon is our fat burning hormone, so we want to encourage its release rather than that of insulin.

With a little forward planning we can help this process work smoothly in order to have maximum time doing nothing (sleeping) while we burn fat. We need about 2.5 to 3 hours from our last meal of the day before we go to bed: so if you go to bed at 10pm (hopefully not later than that for cortisol management) then you need to have dinner at 7pm. For some people this is not easy because work pressures keep them at the office for longer and to arrive home and cook and eat all by 7pm is challenging but it can be done.

Some pre- planning tips
- Shop for vegetables over the weekend. Wash and chop them immediately and place them in small stackable containers in the fridge to be pulled out and steamed. Steaming only takes about 7 minutes.
- Cook your meat dishes in bulk and divide and freeze. If you prepare several meals then it is easy to rotate when you arrive home too late to cook from scratch.
- Prepare sauces for drizzling on your veggies, that will keep for a week in the fridge
- Rice can be pre-prepared and freezes very well although rice at night is not advisable if you are insulin resistant.
- Use herbs with your veggies and rice dishes. Garlic, basil, and thyme are scrumptious

- If you have children, even relatively young children, make them the 'officers- in- charge' of making the salad. Suggest they make rainbow salads finding every colour of the rainbow to put in the food. Strawberries and grapes make a wonderful taste addition to bland salads.

Activity: Shop for the small containers at a thrift ship (glass if you can get). Choose neat and stackable so they will fit well in the refrigerator. At the same time, get your fragrant herbs and spices. Shop with your children so they can smell the different herbs and begin the culinary process towards health. Avoid snacking after dinner.

Day 20

"The only way of finding the limits of the possible is by going beyond them into the impossible." – Arthur C. Clarke

Low carb dinner recipe...

This is a fresh and delicious recipe that is very quick to prepare and tastes fabulous from a delightful site, full of quick and easy recipes that will not spike your blood sugar but will keep your tummy full.
https://alldayidreamaboutfood.com/easy-low-carb-lemongrass-chicken/

Lemongrass Chicken

Cilantro Cauli Rice

2 tbsp avocado oil
1 large head cauliflower, riced (if using pre-riced cauliflower, use 16 ounces)
1/2 tsp salt
1/2 tsp pepper
1 tbsp Lightly Dried Cilantro
Lemongrass Chicken
1 tbsp fish sauce
3 tsp Garlic Paste
1/2 tsp sea salt
1 1/2 lbs. boneless, skinless chicken thighs, cut into 1-inch pieces
2 tbsp xylitol
2 tbsp water, divided
2 tsp molasses
2 tbsp avocado oil
3 tbsp Lemongrass Paste
1 to 2 tsp Lightly Dried Red Chile (more to taste)

Directions
Cauliflower Rice:
Place a medium skillet over medium heat. When hot, add oil and swirl to coat pan. Add rice cauliflower, salt, and pepper and toss to coat in the oil. Cook, stirring frequently, until tender crisp. About 5 minutes.
Add cilantro paste and stir to combine. Cook one minute more, then remove from heat.

Lemongrass Chicken:
In a medium bowl, combine fish sauce, garlic paste and sea salt. Add chicken and toss to combine.
In a small skillet over medium heat, combine sweetener, 1 tbsp water, molasses. Cook, stirring frequently, until sweetener is dissolved. Bring to a boil and cook until mixture is a golden caramel colour. Whisk in remaining water and set aside.

Heat a large wok or skillet over medium high heat. Add oil and swirl to coat. Add lemongrass paste and chili paste and stir until fragrant, about 1 minute.
Add chicken and stir fry until chicken is mostly cooked through, then add caramel mixture and cook until sauce is reduced and thickened.
Serve over cilantro cauliflower rice.

Activity: Make a double batch and freeze half

Day 21

"Many of life's failures are experienced by people who did not realize how close they were to success when they gave up." – Thomas Edison

More herbs for health...

Some herbs, in addition to their unique scent, have medicinal qualities. In this day and age of technology and advanced medicine, we have forgotten that in the past the produce from the rich earth sustained us as well as made us well. Herbs and spices were brewed and steeped to assist in the magical process of giving birth, living well, and dying with dignity. Rosemary, oregano, and sage are three herbs that add a depth to our meals as well as herbs that have beneficial properties to improve sugar management.

Rosemary: Some interesting studies have looked at the effect Rosemary has on blood glucose. Supplementing with Rosemary leaf extract significantly lowered the serum glucose level. This is fantastic news because Rosemary is both delicious and very easy to grow. Even I, with my black fingers, am able to keep my Rosemary bush alive!

Oregano; Contains special compounds called glucosides that have an effect on blood sugars, lowering them in the blood. Oregano is a prolific grower and can grow quite large in a garden. If you are planting in a little planter you need at least 12 inches across to give it some space. Water thoroughly, but let the soil get dry to the touch first.

Sage: In a study published on PubMed, sage was shown to have metformin-like effects on blood sugar. In other words, it lowered serum blood sugar and may help prevent type2 diabetes.
To grow sage you can grow from seeds, but it responds best when you take cuttings from an established plant. Start the plant indoors in the winter and plant in well-drained soil just before summer.

A warning if you already have type 2 diabetes: Adding beneficial herbs that may lower blood glucose may drop your levels too low if you are already on diabetes meds. Please monitor how you feel and chat to your doctor about adjusting your medication. It is always better to reduce the medication rather than eschew the herbs.

Activity: Visit a nursery and after a restful wander around, enjoying the colours and exquisite flowers, buy some herbs and start your herbal health garden

Day 22

"The journey of a thousand miles begins with one step." – Lao Tzu

Benefits of 'high intensity interval training'...

In a busy life it is challenging to get to the gym. I never feel like exercising at the end of the day and in winter, getting up early and in the dark is no fun at all, but there are too many benefits to exercising that I simply cannot ignore.

Fortunately there is a technique called 'high intensity interval training' that works effectively and takes very little time. The advantage when one is struggling with insulin resistance or belly fat is that it can be done anywhere and anytime, and it is very effective in reducing blood sugar. It also helps to increase a hormone called 'human growth hormone' that keeps our muscles dense and in good condition.

There are two ways to approach HIIT. One is to do a 30 second burst of high intensity exercise and rest for 90 seconds. Repeat this 8 times, and the other way is to spread the 30 second bursts throughout the day. The trick is to move hard and fast enough that at the end of the 30 seconds you are panting. This is my program.

- Wake up and run madly on the spot for 30 seconds while I wait for shower to heat up.
- Get to work and run as fast as I can up the stairs to my office.
- Just before lunch run again up the stairs (and down if it's a short flight).

- Get home and put on pumping music and dance with my children.
- 1 hour after dinner (but 2 hours before bed) I do a series of jumping jacks, burpees (sweat) or I skip (a skipping rope skip).

DONE for the day.

When I go to the gym over the weekend, I start with a 4-minute Tabata training. Tabata is like HIIT except it is a 20 second burst and a 10 second rest, repeated 8 times. (Double sweat!)

Ideas for HIIT
- Push-ups
- Jumping jacks or running on the spot.
- Running up and down stairs, optionally carrying a weight. If you don't have a weight then carry a bag of flour or rice
- Squats with optional hand weights or a bag of sugar/rice
- Skipping
- Stair-stepper
- Elliptical machine
- Exercise bike
- Treadmill

Activity: Try out a few high Intensity exercises and decide on one that you think is do-able for you. Stick a post-it reminder on the shower door, the kettle, and any other place you will see at the time you want to do your 30 seconds. It is amazing how easy it is to forget and just climb into the shower. These are habit changes, and we need reminders.

Day 23

"Do not let what you cannot do interfere with what you can do." – John Wooden

Music and health...

In a beautiful study on premature babies, researchers measured their heartbeat as the parents sang lullabies, or the babies were exposed to an ocean disk that mimics the sounds in the womb or a Gato box that mimics heartbeat. While they all slowed the babies' heartbeat and reduced stress, the singing came out best of all.

I particularly love this study because it represents the influence of music in turning our own health around. Music has been shown to improve the immune system as well as reduce stress.

In another study it was found that music actually improved patients response to pain. In something called 'Vibroacoustic Therapy', the patient lies on a mat or bed or sits in a chair embedded with speakers that transmit vibrations at specific computer-generated frequencies that can be heard and felt. Vibroaccoustics have even shown a benefit in people with Parkinson's.

In fact, in the part of the brain called the cerebellum, rhythm is processed, and the frontal lobes interpret the emotional content of the music. Listening to music that is powerful enough to cause that delicious tingle up the spine can light up the brain's reward center in the same way that chocolate does. A great way to help willpower.

This is a fabulous excuse to take some time every day and listen to music. We are not being lazy and doing nothing. We are actively improving our health. Bright cheerful music can change a mood from being down and depressed to upbeat and invigorated and we tend to eat less when we are invigorated and happy.

We have almost limitless access to music of all genres nowadays. It is worth separating the music into playlists that may change a mood. Keep the happy, up-beat music together and set the tone of your day by listening to it in the morning to motivate you and ready you for the challenges at work. Likewise set aside music that feels calming to you to play on the journey home after a long and difficult day at work.

Take note of the message that is in the lyrics. Avoid lyrics that reflect discord and dissention. Although classical music can be glorious, not all people respond well to it, so do not feel that your choice has to be classical or instrumental. This is 'your' playlist and can reflect what stimulates your own emotional trigger.
Have fun choosing. The options are endless.

Activity: Take a few hours one evening and flip through a whole lot of music choices. Save the ones that make you smile or help you feel calmer.

Day 24

Defeat is not bitter unless you swallow it." – Joe Clark

Stock taking...

Retaining large amounts of fairly detailed data takes energy
and if you are reading this book, chances are your energy
started at low ebb. While the daily progress may be wonderful
for that day, putting it all together and remembering the
details in addition to what is required for your own life, can
be onerous.

The experts say it takes 21 days to change a habit and this is
true if we are dedicated over the full time period but I find in
my own life that the onslaught of information, activities,
memories, and duties in my day sap me; Not of my resolve to
make changes but just of the moment-by-moment memory of
what I need to do.
It helps to take stock every now and again, of what I need to
do and what steps I may have forgotten and indeed, what I
am progressing well with.

Summary
- Never eat after dinner
- Eat only three meals a day
- Allow four to six hours between meals
- Go 12-14 hours from dinner to breakfast
- Have a protein-based breakfast
- Eat to full and do not overeat or under eat
- Eat slowly and calmly
- Practice breathing and appreciation before each meal
- Cut out gluten

- Add a good probiotic
- Add 30 seconds of high intensity activity 4 times a day
- Add magnesium to your diet.

Activity: Tick off any activity you have allowed to slip out of your attention. Resolve to address that for the next few days.

Day 25

"Nobody ever wrote down a plan to be broke, fat, lazy, or stupid. Those things are what happen when you don't have a plan." – Larry Winget

Boosting digestion...

As we grow older our digestive ability functions less effectively. The result is more bloating, more heartburn and more discomfort after eating. There are foods we used to enjoy that we can no longer eat and to top it all, many of us are on ant-acids or proton pump inhibitors that make the situation worse long-term because they suppress stomach acid even further.

Our pancreas, the organ that makes insulin, also makes our digestive enzymes. These enzymes break down the bonds between fats and carbohydrates and are really important in facilitating the extraction of necessary vitamins and nutrients necessary for prolonged health and vitality. Poor digestion not only feels uncomfortable but kicks us onto the downward spiral to poor health because our body is just not getting what it needs to functional optimally.

The signs of sub-optimal digestion are:
- Food in your stool
- Constipation
- Diarrhea
- Bloating
- Acne
- Headaches
- Low energy
- Low back pain
- Oily film on stool
- Intolerance to dietary fats

What can we do to augment the pancreas in producing digestive enzymes?
The easiest approach is to supplement with 2 digestive capsules (check they contain lipase for the break- down of dietary fats). However, because money doesn't grow on trees and digestive enzymes cost money, two teaspoons of apple cider vinegar in a little water, just before the meal is also helpful.
Five minutes before your meal, take the digestive enzymes (or the vinegar). This ensures there is augmented digestive capacity waiting in your stomach for the food to land onto it and be thoroughly digested.

Activity: Take 2 digestive enzymes before meals if you suffer from any of the above symptoms

Day 26

"It is not enough to aim, you must hit." – Italian Proverb

Body temperature and health...

I am all for avoiding hospitals and doctors if possible, but maintaining health requires vigilance. When we neglect the daily vigilance, the weeds of poor health become uncontrollable and when we finally look out the window at the overgrown garden, the task of clearing and cleaning has grown disproportionately and is now a huge problem.

The body is the same. The feelings of discomfort creep up and we may attribute them to being stressed at work, or underlying flu, or anything that at that moment, appears reasonable to us and allows us to sweep the unease under the carpet. Firstly because a shift in our body's balance can be worrying and we have enough to bother us without adding that fear as well and secondly because we may have no idea where to begin to reverse the symptoms. Often because they are so vague and nebulous they are difficult to address directly.

Stress is indeed a pervasive problem and interestingly, taking our body temperature for a week can give us valuable information. Our body temp reflects out metabolic activity. A low temp means low metabolic activity and this is fatal if we are trying to shed that belly fat.

Typically an average temp is 98.6 degrees. People who are old and frail may have a temp of between 95-97 degrees. Similarly people who have low thyroid function. Their basal body temp is low because their metabolic rate is too low. If you have a temp of 100 degrees or higher you may either be hyperthyroid (over active thyroid) or be fighting an infection.

The reason we test temperature over a week is because when there is a wide variability of temp then it may indicate adrenal stress. When your adrenals are happy and healthy they project a very even temperature with little variability. First prize is an adequate basal temperature that doesn't vary much.

If your variability is high, take the time over the next few days to meditate, go for massages, take time for yourself, and keep testing your temp. As your adrenals and stress levels calm down, so should the variability on your basal temperature.

Activity: Test and chart your temperature every morning before rising, for a week.

Day 27

"Challenges are what make life interesting and overcoming them is what makes life meaningful." – Joshua J. Marine

A note on Type 1 diabetes...

If type 2 diabetes comes about because of a surplus of insulin and the resultant insulin resistance, how does type 1 diabetes fit in?

Type 1 diabetes used to be known as juvenile diabetes and has since been classified as an auto- immune condition where the immune system attacks the islet cells in the pancreas and prevents the necessary production of insulin. The result is that there is insufficient insulin to carry the glucose into the cells and the glucose accumulates to dangerous levels in the blood, with severe, even life-threatening consequences.

This condition is outside the scope of this book but recent experiments suggest that stopping the autoimmune attack on the islet cells may reduce or even reverse some cases of type 1 diabetes. There is also some evidence that addresses the association with antibodies to wheat proteins as well as casein from dairy. This is important because a gluten and dairy free diet may be very beneficial in reducing the extremity of the impact of type 1 diabetes.

Studies of infants of type 1 diabetic parents demonstrate that feeding gluten to those infants greatly increases the development of autoimmune attack on the infant pancreas (by factors of 5 to 7 times greater risk). *http://members.cox.net/harold.kraus/gluten/anno_symptoms_files/diabetes.htmInflammation can lead to insulin resistance*

Activity: If you have, or know of someone who has, type 1 diabetes, research the impact of dairy and gluten and consider eliminating these from the diet.

Day 28

"Every strike brings me closer to the next home run." – Babe Ruth

Measuring carbohydrate quantities...

If we have to reduce the carbohydrates we eat, how can we manage the changes while we also work in our own industry and manage the needs of our family? It is easier for a person who is in the food industry or the health industry, to calculate the finer details of the carb content of each meal but what if you are in finance, or dressmaking or another profession diametrically opposite to food and health? I find that a bird's eye view helps make choices when we are standing with our empty plate in front of the buffet table.

How many grams of carbohydrates will impact on my health and waistline?

- **0 to 50 grams per day** - This is an extremely low consumption. It is usually the level of carb intake in a ketogenic diet or during a fasting state. This works very well for limited time to bring down fasting insulin swiftly
- **50-100 grams per day**- A manageable range to start to bring down the insulin impact.
- **100 to 150 grams per day**- This is an adequate range to maintain a weight when you are young but as you get older or hit menopause, even this level is a bit high, unless you are an athlete
- **150 to 300 grams per day**- Not beneficial for longevity and insulin management.
- **300 or more grams per day- Dangerous**
-

Examples of Food: **Average**
Carbohydrate in grams
- Teaspoon of sugar
  5 grams

- Small bar of chocolate
  - 50 grams
- All bread, even gluten free bread
  - 16 grams per slice
- Rice
  - 18 grams per ½ cup
- Pasta, even gluten free,
  - 37 grams per cup
- Carrots (cooked)
  - 10 grams per cup
- Potato small
  - 18 grams
- Lentils and beans
  - 21 grams per ½ cup
- Beets
  - 12 grams per cup
- Apple (medium)
  - 18 grams
- Banana (medium)
  - 23 grams
- Watermelon (low GL)
  - 29 grams
- Berries
  - 20 grams
- Grapes
  - 30 grams per cup
- Dried fruit
  - 60 grams per ½ cup
- Vegetables
  - Zero
- Salad
  - Zero

Although the above list is a rough estimate, one can see that if you are re-sensitizing your cells to insulin and want to keep carb levels down, one cheese sandwich and a cup of tea with 1 teaspoon of sugar will add close to 50 grams of carbohydrate. That is your whole daily allowance gone!
Whereas a large salad with nuts an avocado, adds hardly any carbs to your daily allowance.

Activity: Check the carbohydrate content of the foods you love using 'Cronometer' or another app and take note of the quantity you can eat to make little impact on daily Carbohydrate load.

Day 29

"I am not a product of my circumstances. I am a product of my decisions." – Stephen Covey

Treats. More treats...

I need treats. Often! Treats help me deal with stress and prevent me from becoming rigid and sour in my approach to life. Being rigid is unlikable as well as ungenerous. I have friends who are naturally indulgent and generous, both with their time and their energy but oftentimes are also a tad too generous with the indulgencies they allow themselves; - of all the most damaging sorts.
I try to balance that indulgence by allowing myself treats but being careful they will not impact negatively on my health.

The following recipe is delicious and I love the title of the website.
https://alldayidreamaboutfood.com/low-carb-no-bake-chocolate-mousse-tart/

Chocolate mousse tart

Ingredients
Crust

- 1 1/4 cups **almond flour**
- 1/4 cup **cocoa powder**
- 1/4 cup **powdered Swerve Sweetener**
- 5 tbsp butter, melted
- Chocolate Mousse Filling
- 3/4 cup whipping cream
- 3/4 cup unsweetened almond or cashew milk
- 1/4 cup butter
- 3 ounces **good quality unsweetened dark chocolate**, chopped (do not use sweetened chocolate here, as your mousse may not set properly)
- 3 tbsp **cocoa powder**
- 6 tbsp **powdered Swerve Sweetener**
- 1/2 tsp **espresso powder** (optional, boosts chocolate flavour)
- 3 large eggs*

Topping

- 1 cup whipping cream
- 2 tbsp **powdered Swerve Sweetener**
- 1/4 tsp **vanilla extract**
- 1/2 ounce **dark sugar-free chocolate**

Directions
Crust:
Lightly grease a 9-inch tart pan with a removable bottom.

In a medium bowl, whisk together the almond flour, cocoa powder, and sweetener. Add melted butter and stir until the mixture clumps together.
Press firmly and evenly into bottom and up sides of prepared tart pan. Refrigerate until filling is ready.

Chocolate Mousse:
In a small pan, combine cream, almond or cashew milk, and butter. Bring to a full boil and then remove from heat.
In a blender, combine unsweetened chocolate, cocoa powder, sweetener, and espresso powder. Pour in scalded cream mixture and blend until smooth.
Add eggs and blend again until smooth (*if you are concerned about the eggs, use pasteurized shell eggs such as Safest Choice). Pour into chilled crust and chill until firm, at least 1 hour. Gently press the tart pan from the bottom to remove the sides and place on a serving platter.

Topping:
Beat whipping cream with sweetener and vanilla until it holds stiff peaks. Spread over mousse to the edges of the tart.
Using a cheese grater, shave the dark chocolate over the whipping cream. Let set a bit in the refrigerator before serving.
by **Carolyn**

Recipe Notes
Serves 12. Each serving has 3.91 g NET CARBS.
Food energy: 359kcal Total fat: 33.46g Calories from fat: 301 Cholesterol: 122mg Carbohydrate: 7.95g Total dietary fiber: 4.04g Protein: 6.64g

Activity: Make this delicious treat and indulge when you are feeling low and need to spoil yourself.

Day 30

Hidden dangers to health...

The food industry is here to make money. They are not concerned with your health and certainly not concerned with your image. The result of this is that processed food is carefully combined to stimulate the pleasure centres in the brain so that you will keep coming back for more.

Gluten and sugar as well as damaging trans-fats, are hidden under names we do not recognise and when we are struggling with our health it is helpful to know where they hide so we can avoid those foods. Of course, the most obvious guideline is to eat food that actually looks like the real deal. Cereals do not grow on trees and shopping in the fresh produce side of the supermarket will eliminate any hidden dangers but because we are busy and occasionally need a quick convenient snack, the following list will illustrate what to watch out for.

<u>Hidden Sugar</u>
Baby Foods (truly)
Biscuits, Breads
Cakes
Candies
Cereals and instant oats
Chocolate (Duh)
Cocoa Drinks
Cookies
Crackers
Custards, Puddings
Doughnuts
Frosting and icing
Ice Cream, Sherbets
Lunch Meats
Marshmallows
Macaroons
Mayonnaise
Meringues
Pancakes, Waffles
Processed Foods
Salad Dressings
Sauces
Soft Drinks

Soups   Wheat Germ, Bran
Sorbets
Yogurt. Flavoured

Hidden Gluten
Beer, Alcohol
Biscuits, Rolls
Breads:
 Crumbed Fish or chicken
Crumbed Meats
Wheat, Rye, Oat,
Spelt, Pumpernickel
Bouillon and stock Cubes
Cakes, Muffins
Candy, Chocolates
Cereals and muesli
Crackers
Cocoa Drinks
Cookies, Pretzels
Cooked Meat Dishes
Corn Bread, Muffins
Crackers
Doughnuts, Popovers
Dumplings and gnocchi
Flour:
White, Wheat
Gravies
Matzos
Packaged Mixes
Pancakes, Waffles
Pasta, Noodles
Pie Crust
Ovaltine
Soufflés
Soy Sauce
Tamari

Activity: Remove from your pantry any of the foods that have hidden gluten or sugar. Check labels of the foods you love.

Day 31

"We become what we think about." – Earl Nightingale

My 'Start' Journal...

Even slim people may have insulin resistance despite the fact they have no belly fat. Although how we look and feel is very often an indication of what is going on at a cellular level and - just as we have our car serviced on a yearly basis, peeking beneath the hood of our body is advisable on a yearly basis and blood tests are the way to do this, as well as a review of how we feel.

Look back to and blood tests you had done previously and jot down any that are related to insulin resistance and how our body manages sugars. Keeping these within optimal range as we age, will keep us vital and energetic.

I also think it is a great idea to take a 'before' photo. I admire the many people who post the before and after photo's on Instagram. I am not that brave but I want to applaud madly when I see some of the remarkable changes effort can bring about. Well done to all these people and well done to you, my reader, as you embark on your own quest for 'slim and vital'. **Record the before and after:**

Weight	
HBA1c	
Fasting Glucose	
Fasting Insulin	
Hs-CRP	
Photo	

Activity: Take note of your vitals today and then again in 3 months.

You:
- Addressed whether you have some signs of insulin resistance
- Delved into a greater understanding of how insulin works in the body
- Began to understand where the body gets energy while sleeping
- Took note of your own eating patterns

- Addressed your HBA1c again to see where you stand with regard to insulin resistance
- Measured your blood pressure
- Tried out some yummy recipes
- Began belly breathing to reduce stress
- Addressed other causes for insulin resistance in your own life
- Reduced obstacles to your own good night's rest
- Added water to your daily activities
- Added important supplements like magnesium, chromium, and omega 3
- Addressed the GL , or GI, of foods you love
- Removed plastic from part of my daily habits such as my water bottle
- Added protein to every meal, especially breakfast
- Cut out some particularly unhealthy drinks or meals from my daily activities
- Bought a glucometer to track my food
- Aimed to go 4-5 hours between meals with no snacking
- Prepared my kitchen and shopped for advanced cooking
- Started an herb garden with rosemary, sage, and oregano
- Added 30 seconds of high intensity activity to my day
- Sorted out my playlists
- Added digestive support to my meals
- Took my temperature for a week to assess my stress levels
- Monitored the carbohydrate quantities of the foods I particularly love
- Evaluated my pantry for hidden gluten and sugars
- Started my before and after journal